GAO

Report to the Ranking Member,
Committee on the Judiciary, U.S.
Senate

August 2012

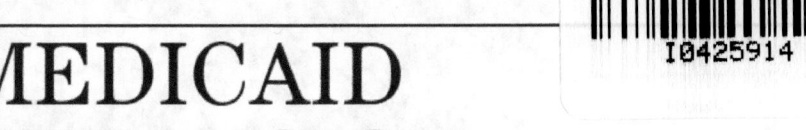

I0425914

MEDICAID EXPANSION

States' Implementation of the Patient Protection and Affordable Care Act

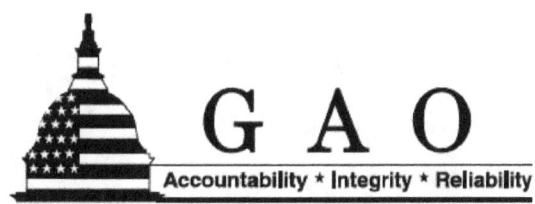

GAO

Accountability * Integrity * Reliability

Contents

Figures

Abbreviations

CHIP	Children's Health Insurance Program
CMS	Centers for Medicare & Medicaid Services
FPL	federal poverty level
FMAP	Federal Medical Assistance Percentage
HCERA	Health Care and Education Reconciliation Act
HHS	Department of Health and Human Services
MAGI	Modified Adjusted Gross Income
PPACA	Patient Protection and Affordable Care Act

View GAO-12-944SP Key Components

Medicaid Expansion: States' Implementation of the Patient Protection and Affordable Care Act (GAO-12-944SP), an e-supplement to GAO-12-821.

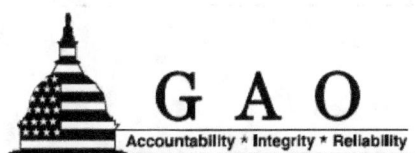

United States Government Accountability Office
Washington, DC 20548

August 1, 2012

The Honorable Charles E. Grassley
Ranking Member
Committee on the Judiciary
United States Senate

Dear Senator Grassley:

The Patient Protection and Affordable Care Act (PPACA), signed into law
on March 23, 2010, made significant changes to the way eligibility for the
Medicaid program will be determined and who the program will cover.[1]
Under PPACA, eligibility for Medicaid—a joint federal-state program that
finances health care for certain categories of low-income individuals—
must be expanded to non-elderly individuals with incomes at or below 133
percent of the federal poverty level (FPL) beginning on January 1,
2014.[2,3] Through this expansion, states will provide Medicaid coverage to
eligible low-income parents and childless adults. PPACA also requires the
establishment of American Health Benefit Exchanges (referred to as
exchanges)—marketplaces where eligible individuals can purchase

---

[1] Pub. L. No. 111-148, 124 Stat. 119 (Mar. 23, 2010) (PPACA), as amended by the Health
Care and Education Reconciliation Act, Pub. L. No. 111-152, 124 Stat. 1029 (Mar. 30,
2010).

[2] PPACA § 2001(a)(1),124 Stat. 271. In this report, we refer to this group as the "newly
eligible." We use FPL to refer to federal poverty guidelines issued by the Department of
Health and Human Services each year in the *Federal Register*. These guidelines provide
income thresholds that vary by family size and for certain states, and which are updated
using the Consumer Price Index. The national Medicaid minimum eligibility level of 133
percent of FPL was $29,700 for a family of four in 2011.

[3] Under the Medicaid program, a failure by a state to comply with federal requirements
may result in a termination of federal Medicaid funds by the Secretary of Health and
Human Services. 42 U.S.C. § 1396c. The U.S. Supreme Court recently ruled that any
state that chooses not to expand Medicaid coverage to the newly eligible will not be
subject to this penalty. Instead, the state will forego the enhanced federal matching funds
associated with covering this population. See *National Federation of Independent
Business, et al., vs. Sebelius, Sec. of Health and Human Services, et al.*, 567 U.S._, 2012
WL 2427810 (U.S. June 28, 2012).

private health insurance in each state.[4] The Centers for Medicare & Medicaid Services' (CMS) Office of the Actuary has estimated that, as a result of the expansion, the number of Medicaid enrollees will increase by 14.9 million in 2014 and by 25.9 million in 2020.[5]

State governments will play a key role in implementing many aspects of this reform, which must be in place by the beginning of 2014. Specifically, states will need to make major changes to the way they conduct Medicaid eligibility determinations for individuals and families. States also will need to develop streamlined eligibility and enrollment systems that allow for the coordination of enrollment across Medicaid, the Children's Health Insurance Program (CHIP),[6] and exchanges. At the same time, states will need to address the financial implications of implementing this Medicaid expansion and accompanying enrollment systems. The federal government will initially provide states with full funding to cover the cost of adults who are newly eligible for Medicaid due to the expansion.

You asked us to report on the actions states are taking to implement the Medicaid expansion. This report addresses the following questions:

1. What are states' responsibilities for implementing the Medicaid expansion provisions under PPACA?

---

[4]PPACA requires the establishment of exchanges in each state by January 1, 2014. PPACA § 1311(b), 124 Stat. 173. Through each state's exchange, individuals can compare and select insurance coverage from among participating health insurance plans. PPACA § 1312, 124 Stat. 182-183. Premium tax credits and cost sharing reductions for these plans will be available for eligible individuals or families with income from 100 to 400 percent of the FPL. PPACA §§ 1401(a),1402 124 Stat. 213-24, as amended by HCERA § 1001, 124 Stat. 1030-32. In addition, if a state does not elect to operate an exchange, the Secretary of the Department of Health and Human Services, either directly or through an agreement with a nonprofit entity, will establish and operate an exchange within that state. PPACA § 1321(c), 124 Stat. 186-7.

[5]Office of the Actuary, Centers for Medicare & Medicaid Services, *United States Department of Health & Human Services: 2011 Actuarial Report on the Financial Outlook for Medicaid* (Mar. 16, 2012).

[6]CHIP is a federal-state program and provides health care coverage to children 18 years of age and younger living in low-income families whose incomes exceed the eligibility requirements for Medicaid.

2. What actions have selected states taken to prepare for the Medicaid expansion provisions of PPACA and what challenges have they encountered?

3. What are states' views on the fiscal implications of the Medicaid expansion on state budget planning?

To identify states' responsibilities for implementing the Medicaid expansion, we reviewed selected PPACA provisions (see table 1).

Table 1: Description of Selected Provisions of PPACA Included in Our Review

PPACA provision	Description
Medicaid eligibility expansion	States must expand Medicaid eligibility to non-elderly individuals with incomes at or below 133 percent of the federal poverty level. Through this expansion, states will provide Medicaid coverage to newly eligible low-income parents and childless adults.
Transition to modified adjusted gross income (MAGI)	States must begin determining income eligibility for Medicaid beneficiaries using a uniform methodology—modified adjusted gross income.
Medicaid early expansion option	States may choose to expand coverage to those newly eligible prior to January 1, 2014.
Maintenance of effort requirement	States must maintain its Medicaid eligibility standards until an exchange in the state is fully operational.
Increased federal matching rates for newly eligible adults	States will receive an increased federal match for newly eligible adults at 100 percent for 2014 through 2016 and gradually decreasing to 90 percent by 2020.
Streamlined eligibility and enrollment systems	States must provide a process for individuals to apply for or renew their Medicaid eligibility through a website that enrolls individuals in the appropriate program (Medicaid, CHIP, or exchanges) no matter to which program they originally apply.

Source: GAO review of PPACA.

We also reviewed the implementing regulations and guidance from CMS, the agency within the Department of Health and Human Services (HHS) that oversees states' Medicaid programs at the federal level. During interviews with CMS officials, we obtained status updates on the development of additional regulations and guidance and discussed the ways CMS provided implementation information to states. We also discussed the implementation of these provisions with selected states.

To identify the actions selected states have taken to prepare for the implementation of the Medicaid expansion and the challenges they encountered, we conducted semi-structured interviews with state Medicaid officials in six states: Colorado, Georgia, Iowa, Minnesota, New York, and Virginia. We selected these states on the basis of: (1) the relative size of expected enrollment expansion within Medicaid, (2) the state's Medicaid enrollment rates, (3) geographic dispersion, and (4) whether a state expanded insurance coverage to childless adults in the past. The findings from these interviews cannot be generalized to all state Medicaid offices. We obtained additional information from interviews with officials from state associations, including the National Association of Medicaid Directors, the National Association of State Budget Officers, and the National Conference of State Legislatures.

To identify states' views on the fiscal implications of the Medicaid expansion on state budget planning, we administered a web-based survey of state budget directors from all 50 states, the District of Columbia, and 4 U.S. territories. Our survey response rate was 76 percent. The survey document and counts of responses received for each question are reproduced in an e-supplement we are issuing concurrent with this report—GAO-12-944SP.[7] To obtain additional narrative and supporting context, survey respondents were given multiple opportunities to provide additional open-ended comments throughout our survey. To limit possible data processing errors, survey response data were checked for inconsistencies and ineligible responses. We also obtained additional information from interviews with federal and state officials and relevant state associations. For more details on our scope and methodology, see appendix IV.

We conducted our work from June 2011 to July 2012 in accordance with generally accepted government audit standards. Those standards require that we plan and perform the audit to obtain sufficient, appropriate evidence to provide a reasonable basis for our findings and conclusions based on our audit objectives. We believe that the evidence obtained, and the analysis conducted, provides a reasonable basis for our findings and conclusions based on our audit objectives.

---

[7]GAO, *E: supplement: Medicaid Expansion: States' Implementation of the Patient Protection and Affordable Care Act*, GAO-12-944SP (Washington, D.C.: Aug.1, 2012).

We completed our field work prior to the U.S. Supreme Court's June 28, 2012, decision on the constitutionality of certain PPACA provisions, including the Medicaid expansion provision discussed in this analysis.[8] Given the timing of the court's decision, and the completion of our field work, we do not include an analysis of the impact of this decision.

Background

Medicaid is a joint federal-state program that provides health care coverage for certain low-income individuals. At the federal level, CMS is responsible for overseeing the design and operation of states' Medicaid programs. States administer their respective Medicaid programs' day-to-day operations within federal requirements. To receive federal matching dollars for services provided to Medicaid beneficiaries each state must submit a state Medicaid plan for consideration, review, and approval by CMS.[9]

Medicaid is funded jointly by the federal government and states. The amount of federal funds states receive is determined by a statutory formula—the Federal Medical Assistance Percentage (FMAP). Under the FMAP, the federal government pays a share of Medicaid expenditures based on each state's per capita income relative to the national average. The FMAP for federal fiscal year 2012 for states ranged from about 50 percent to 74 percent. According to the National Governors Association and the National Association of State Budget Officers spring 2012 survey, Medicaid represents the largest portion of total state spending, accounting for an estimated 23 percent of state spending in fiscal year 2011.[10]

Under federal Medicaid law, states generally must meet certain minimum requirements for establishing eligibility for individuals. Eligibility for Medicaid is based on a variety of categorical and financial requirements. For example, Medicaid eligibility focuses on parents and children, individuals who are aged, and individuals with disabilities. Additionally, individuals who are eligible for Medicaid must have limited income and

---

[8]*National Federation of Independent Business, et al., vs. Sebelius, Sec. of Health and Human Services, et al.*, No. 11-393.

[9]A Medicaid state plan describes the scope of a state's Medicaid program, including a list of eligibility categories and standards and the services covered.

[10]National Governors Association and the National Association of State Budget Officers, *The Fiscal Survey of States* (Washington, D.C.: Spring 2012).

resources, and must meet immigration and residency requirements. State-to-state variation in Medicaid eligibility levels exists, particularly for low-income adults. According to the Kaiser Family Foundation, as of January 1, 2012, the median Medicaid eligibility threshold for working parents is 63 percent of FPL and 17 states limit Medicaid coverage to parents earning less than 50 percent of FPL. Rules for counting income to determine eligibility vary from state to state, and can also vary by population within a state.

Summary of Findings

In summary, we found:

- Under PPACA, states are responsible for making a number of changes to their Medicaid programs by January 1, 2014, including expanding eligibility levels and streamlining their enrollment processes. Specifically, states must expand Medicaid eligibility to non-elderly individuals with incomes at or below 133 percent of FPL.[11,12] Under the newly eligible category, states will provide Medicaid coverage to eligible low-income parents and childless adults. States must also begin determining income eligibility for Medicaid beneficiaries, including newly eligible adults, using a uniform methodology—MAGI, which is a tax-based definition of income.[13] To implement these requirements, eligibility categories have been consolidated into four groups—adults, children, parents, and pregnant women. States may choose to expand Medicaid coverage to the newly eligible prior to January 1, 2014 (referred to as the early expansion option), but must cover lower income individuals before higher income individuals. These more uniform eligibility requirements will replace the current system where Medicaid eligibility and income rules may vary from state to state. Further, states must adopt a

---

[11]States must expand Medicaid coverage to non-pregnant individuals who are under 65, who have household incomes at or below 133 percent of the federal poverty level for the applicable family size who are not entitled to or enrolled in Medicare, and who are not already required to be covered under Medicaid.

[12]PPACA also specifies that an income disregard in the amount of 5 percent FPL be deducted from an individual's income when determining Medicaid eligibility. This income counting rule effectively raises the upper income eligibility threshold for new eligibly Medicaid recipients to 138 percent FPL.

[13]Certain groups of individuals are exempt from this requirement, such as individuals who qualify for Medicaid on the basis of being aged, blind, or disabled, and their eligibility will continue to be determined based on existing criteria.

methodology for identifying the newly eligible in order to obtain the increased federal match. States will receive the enhanced federal match for newly eligible adults starting in 2014.[14] States must also provide a simplified and streamlined eligibility process whereby individuals, through a website, may apply for and, if eligible, be enrolled in Medicaid. In addition, state eligibility determination systems will interface with a Federal Data Services Hub—an electronic service states will use to verify certain information with other federal agencies, such as an applicant's citizenship, immigration status, and income data. For additional information on our findings, see appendix I.

- The six selected states included in our study (Colorado, Georgia, Iowa, Minnesota, New York, and Virginia) are taking some steps to prepare for the Medicaid expansion, including assessing changes that need to be made to their existing eligibility levels and eligibility determination policies. In an effort to streamline their eligibility and enrollment processes, the six states also are taking steps to upgrade or replace their Medicaid information technology systems and have submitted applications to CMS for enhanced federal funding for this purpose.[15] In our interviews with selected states, officials noted that the enhanced funding provides the states with an opportunity to update outdated eligibility and enrollment systems. At the same time, state officials reported challenges to implementing PPACA's Medicaid expansion requirements, including the need for additional federal regulations and guidance in a number of areas. For example, state officials indicated that they need additional guidance on using MAGI[16] to determine an applicant's eligibility under different scenarios

---

[14]The federal government will pay 100 percent of the cost of covering new eligible individuals in fiscal years 2014, 2015, and 2016, with the federal match gradually reduced to 90 percent by 2020.

[15]The Secretary of Health and Human Services is authorized to provide enhanced administrative funding at a rate of 90 percent of the cost for the design, development, or installation of information technology enrollment systems that are likely to provide more efficient, economical, and effective administration, and 75 percent for the operation of those systems. CMS issued a final rule on April 19, 2011, providing for enhanced funding through December 31, 2015, for states to upgrade their information technology systems to implement the improvements and changes to Medicaid enrollment under PPACA provided that the systems meet a number of standards and conditions.

[16]As stated earlier, MAGI is the new methodology that states will use beginning in 2014 to calculate an applicant's income to determine whether or not they are eligible for Medicaid.

GAO-12-821 Medicaid Expansion

involving household income levels, sources of income, and household composition. CMS has issued a final Medicaid rule[17] and hosted webinars on this and other issues, and said that additional guidance is forthcoming. States also reported operational challenges that could affect their ability to meet Medicaid expansion and system development deadlines, such as lengthy state procurement processes, the complexities of developing new systems, coordination of multiple programs and systems, and resource limitations. For additional information on our findings, see appendix II.

- In terms of states' views on the fiscal implications of the Medicaid expansion on states' budget planning, our survey found that across fiscal years 2012 to 2020, the majority of state budget directors believe that three aspects of Medicaid expansion will contribute to costs: (1) the administration for managing Medicaid enrollment, (2) the acquisition or modification of information technology systems to support Medicaid, and (3) enrolling previously eligible but not enrolled individuals in Medicaid. At the same time, state budget directors expressed uncertainty about how other aspects of expansion will affect their budgets, such as the impact of shifting existing Medicaid enrollees into health benefit exchanges. Further, most state budget directors reported that their fiscal capacity and the state's share of Medicaid expenditures create challenges for implementing the Medicaid expansion. A few state budget directors reported that CMS guidance was useful, while most commented that more guidance was needed to develop budget estimates in the following areas: Medicaid benefits packages (including essential and benchmark benefits), Medicaid eligibility determination, and the FMAP match for newly eligible adults. CMS officials indicated that the agency is planning to issue additional guidance or regulations at a later date in a number of areas, including clarification on eligibility groups, MAGI, and the FMAP methodology for the newly eligible population. For additional detail on our findings, see appendix III.

---

[17]CMS, *Medicaid Program; Eligibility Changes Under the Affordable Care Act of 2010,* Final Rule and Interim Final Rule, 77 Fed. Reg. 17,144 (Washington, D.C.: Mar. 23, 2012).

Concluding Observations

It has been a little over 2 years since the enactment of PPACA, which included significant changes to the Medicaid program. The ultimate success of the implementation of these changes will depend heavily on both federal and state actions. States reported needing additional federal regulations or guidance in three areas: application of MAGI methodology, conversion of Medicaid eligibility standards, and eligibility data available to states through the Federal Data Services Hub. According to state officials, the release of regulations or guidance could affect their state's ability to meet implementation deadlines. CMS issued regulations and guidance on a range of topics regarding Medicaid expansion and has indicated that additional guidance will be forthcoming. Concerted and cooperative efforts on the part of CMS and the states will be critical to meeting the implementation deadlines for the Medicaid expansion.

Agency Comments and Our Evaluation

We provided the draft for review and comment to HHS. HHS provided us with written comments and agreed with our conclusion that additional regulations or guidance is needed in various areas, such as MAGI conversion and the computation of FMAP. HHS said it plans to issue such guidance later this year. It also noted that our report was a helpful resource for purposes of targeting its ongoing technical assistance implementation efforts with states and outlined several areas in which additional guidance or technical assistance will be forthcoming. Regarding the Supreme Court's June 28, 2012, decision that states can make their own decisions about whether to expand Medicaid, HHS reiterated that (1) there is no deadline for a state to decide to undertake the expansion; (2) a state can receive enhanced administrative federal match for information technology costs, even if it has not yet decided whether to expand Medicaid, as long as it is modernizing its eligibility systems; and (3) a state will not have to pay back the extra funding if it ultimately decides not to expand Medicaid. HHS's written comments are reproduced in appendix V. Additionally, we provided excerpts of the draft report to officials in the six states we interviewed for this study and incorporated their technical comments as appropriate.

We are sending copies of this report to the appropriate congressional committees and other interested parties. The report is also available at no charge on the GAO website at http://www.gao.gov.

If you have any questions concerning this report, please contact Stanley J. Czerwinski at (202) 512-6806 or czerwinskis@gao.gov or Carolyn L. Yocom at (202) 512-7114 or yocomc@gao.gov. Contact points for our Offices of Congressional Relations and Public Affairs may be found on the last page of this report. Key contributors to this report are listed in appendix VI.

Sincerely yours,

Stanley J. Czerwinski
Director
Strategic Issues

Carolyn L. Yocom
Director, Health Care

Appendix I: States Must Expand Medicaid Eligibility Levels and Streamline the Enrollment Process

Under the Patient Protection and Affordable Care Act, States Must Expand Medicaid Eligibility Levels and Streamline the Enrollment Process

As of January 1, 2014, states must (1) expand Medicaid eligibility to non-elderly individuals with incomes at or below 133 percent of the federal poverty level (FPL)[1,2] and (2) begin determining income eligibility for Medicaid beneficiaries, including those newly eligible, using a uniform methodology—modified adjusted gross income (MAGI),[3] a tax-based definition of income. Prior to January 1, 2014, states may choose to expand eligibility to those newly eligible (referred to as the early expansion option),[4] but must cover lower income individuals before higher income individuals.

Under the newly eligible category, states will provide Medicaid coverage to eligible low-income parents and childless adults. In addition, these more uniform national requirements will replace the current system where Medicaid eligibility and income rules may vary from state to state. Currently under Medicaid, eligibility is based on a variety of categorical and financial requirements. For example, states must cover certain population groups, such as low-income children and pregnant women, but have flexibility to cover other groups, such as those same groups at higher income levels. Subject to federal minimum standards for income, states also have some flexibility in determining how to calculate income, such as by excluding certain types of income (e.g., child support payments) or applying asset tests (e.g., value of an automobile). Under

---

[1]PPACA § 2001(a)(1), 124 Stat. 271. States must expand Medicaid coverage to non-pregnant individuals who are under 65, who have household incomes at or below 133 percent of FPL for the applicable family size, who are not entitled to or enrolled in Medicare, and who are not already required to be covered under Medicaid. In this section, we refer to this group as the "newly eligible."

[2]Under the Medicaid program, a failure by a state to comply with federal requirements may result in a termination of federal Medicaid funds by the Secretary of Health and Human Services. 42 U.S.C. § 1396c. The U.S. Supreme Court recently ruled that any state that chooses not to expand Medicaid coverage to the newly eligible will not be subject to this penalty. Instead, the state will forego the enhanced federal matching funds associated with covering this population. See National Federation of Independent Business, et al., vs. Sebelius, Sec. of Health and Human Services, et al., 567 U.S._, 2012 WL 2427810 (U.S. June 28, 2012).

[3]PPACA § 2002, 124 Stat. 279-82, as amended by the HCERA §§ 1004(b),(e), 124 Stat. 1034, 1036. MAGI, is adjusted gross income, plus certain excluded foreign income and tax-exempt interest. See 26 U.S.C. § 36B(d)(2)(B). Certain groups of individuals are exempt from this requirement, such as individuals who qualify for Medicaid on the basis of being aged, blind, or disabled.

[4]PPACA § 2001(a)(4), 124 Stat. 274, as amended by PPACA § 10201(b), 124 Stat. 918.

GAO-12-821 Medicaid Expansion

the Patient Protection and Affordable Care Act (PPACA), however, states must uniformly cover all eligible individuals at or below 133 percent of the FPL and apply one income methodology using MAGI. To implement these provisions, the Centers for Medicare & Medicaid (CMS) has consolidated these individuals into four groups—adults, children, parents, and pregnant women.[5]

To make their current policies and processes consistent with these new coverage and income eligibility rules, state officials stated they will need to take legislative or regulatory action, and will need to receive federal approval for these changes from CMS. In addition, states' continued receipt of federal matching funds is contingent upon meeting PPACA's maintenance of effort requirement. In particular, states may not make any changes to their Medicaid eligibility levels, methodologies, and procedures for adults that are more restrictive than those in place at the time of PPACA's enactment (Mar. 23, 2010) until the Secretary of the Department of Health and Human Services (HHS) determines that an exchange in the state[6] is fully operational.[7]

States Must Adopt a Methodology to Claim the Increased Federal Match for the Newly Eligible

In order to determine which beneficiaries are newly eligible and which are not, states must evaluate Medicaid applicants against the state's pre-PPACA eligibility rules. States will receive an increased federal match for newly eligible adults at 100 percent for 2014 through 2016, 95 percent in 2017, 94 percent in 2018, 93 percent in 2019, and 90 percent in 2020 and beyond.[8] In general, states that had already covered parents and

---

[5]CMS, *Medicaid Program; Eligibility Changes Under the Affordable Care Act of 2010*, Final Rule and Interim Final Rule, 77 Fed. Reg. 17,144, 17,204-5 (Mar. 23, 2012).

[6]PPACA requires the establishment of a system of American Health Benefit Exchanges—marketplaces where eligible individuals can purchase private health insurance. PPACA § 1311(b),124 Stat. 173. Through each state's exchange, individuals can compare and select insurance coverage from amongst participating health insurance plans. PPACA § 1312, 124 Stat. 182-3.

[7]PPACA § 2001(b)(1)-(3), 124 Stat. 275-76. PPACA also requires states to maintain Medicaid eligibility levels for children from March 23, 2010, through September 30, 2019. Exceptions to maintenance of effort requirements may be granted for Medicaid eligibility restrictions for non-pregnant, non-disabled adults with income above 133 percent of the federal poverty level for states experiencing or projecting a budget deficit.

[8]PPACA §§ 2001(a)(3),124 Stat. 272-3, as amended by PPACA §10201(c)(3)(B),124 Stat. 918-19 and HCERA § 1201(1)(B),124 Stat. 1051-52.

childless adults with incomes of at least 100 percent FPL prior to PPACA may receive an increased federal match starting in 2014 for covering these individuals.[9]

States Must Simplify and Streamline Medicaid Enrollment Processes

By January 1, 2014, states must provide a process whereby individuals, through a website, may apply for or renew their eligibility for Medicaid.[10] States must also participate in a coordinated eligibility and enrollment process for Medicaid and other health insurance programs, including the Children's Health Insurance Program (CHIP) and the health insurance exchanges.[11] The systems for these programs are required to work together to ensure that eligible applicants are enrolled in the appropriate program no matter to which program they originally apply—referred to as the "no wrong door" policy. For each individual not eligible for Medicaid based on MAGI, the eligibility system will collect additional information to determine eligibility based on other factors.

In addition, state eligibility determination systems will interface with a Federal Data Services Hub (referred to as the federal hub). The federal hub is an electronic service under development by HHS that states will use to verify certain information with other federal agencies, such as an applicant's citizenship through the Social Security Administration, immigration status through the Department of Homeland Security, and income data through the Internal Revenue Service. States may receive an enhanced administrative federal match—90 percent—for the design,

---

[9]PPACA § 10201(c), 124 Stat. 918-19, as amended by HCERA § 1201, 124 Stat. 1051-2. These states are eligible for an increased federal matching rate for this population based on a formula that will vary based on their regular Federal Medical Assistance Percentage until calendar year 2019, at which point they will receive the newly eligible federal matching rate described earlier.

[10]PPACA makes this requirement a condition for the receipt of federal funding for states' Medicaid programs.

[11]PPACA § 2201, 124 Stat. 289-91. For example, PPACA requires that individuals who are determined ineligible for Medicaid or CHIP be screened for eligibility for the health insurance exchanges. Those that are uninsured with incomes from 100 to 400 percent of the FPL may qualify for premium tax credits and cost sharing reductions for insurance purchased through an exchange.

development, and installation or enhancement of eligibility determination systems until December 31, 2015.[12]

CMS Has Published Implementing Regulations and Guidance

CMS published a final Medicaid eligibility rule on March 23, 2012, to implement certain PPACA requirements.[13] In finalizing the Medicaid eligibility rule, CMS considered public comments on the proposed Medicaid eligibility rule issued in August 17, 2011. The final Medicaid eligibility rule addresses the following: (1) expanding eligibility to adults with incomes at or below 133 percent FPL, (2) applying MAGI for income determination and clarifying MAGI exclusions such as individuals with disabilities and those needing long-term care, and (3) streamlining eligibility screening and enrollment. CMS held conference calls and webinars after issuing the proposed regulation and final rule to provide further clarification to states. See figure 1 for a timeline of the Medicaid provisions and milestones under PPACA described in this appendix.

---

[12]In order to qualify for this enhanced funding, CMS must determine that a state's system meets a number of standards and conditions, including seamless coordination with the exchanges. The 90 percent match is available only for these costs that are incurred from April 19, 2011, through December 31, 2015.

[13]CMS, *Medicaid Program; Eligibility Changes Under the Affordable Care Act of 2010*, Final Rule and Interim Final Rule, 77 Fed. Reg. 17,144 (Mar. 23, 2012).

Figure 1: Timeline for Selected PPACA Provisions

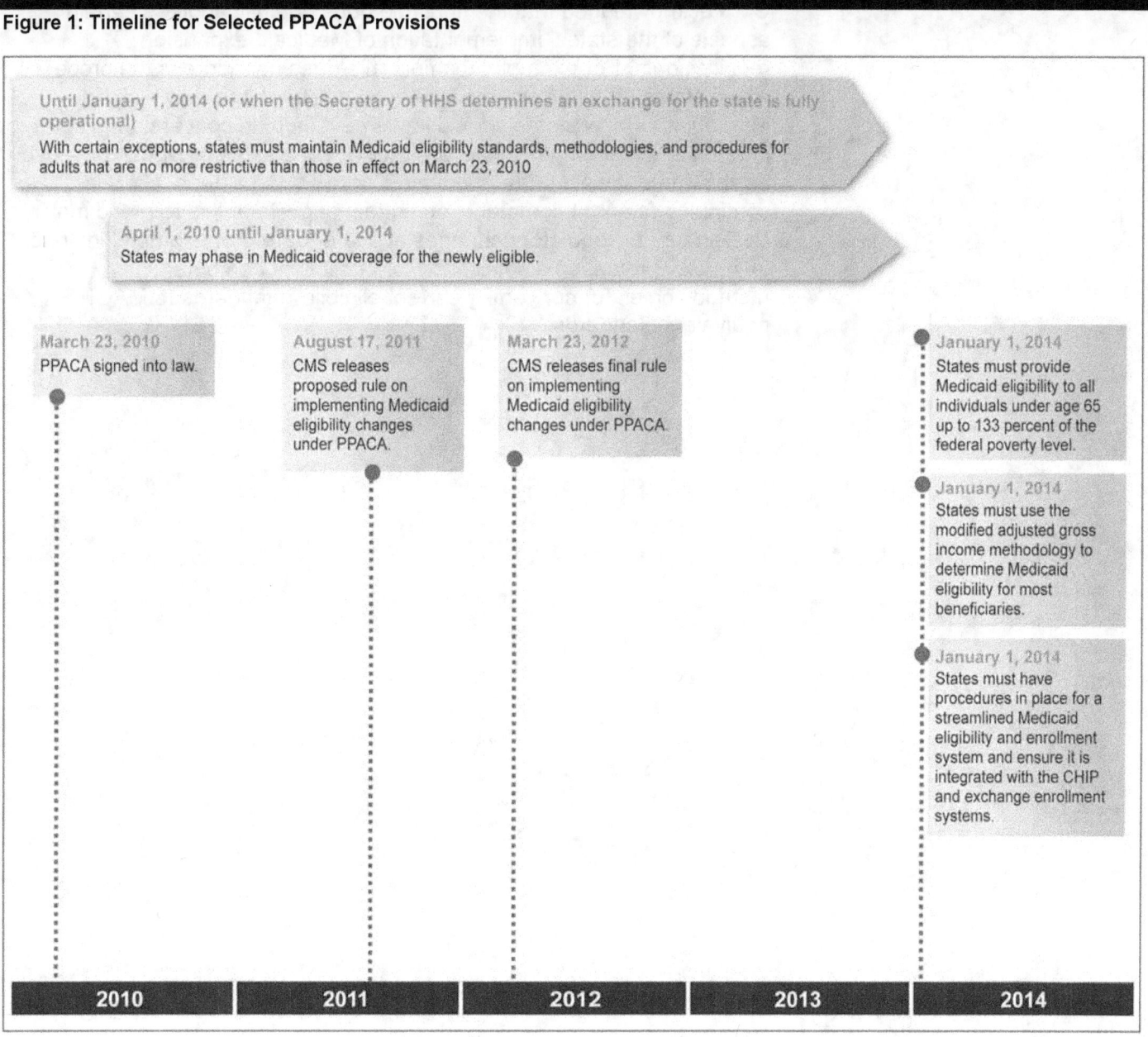

Until January 1, 2014 (or when the Secretary of HHS determines an exchange for the state is fully operational)

With certain exceptions, states must maintain Medicaid eligibility standards, methodologies, and procedures for adults that are no more restrictive than those in effect on March 23, 2010

April 1, 2010 until January 1, 2014

States may phase in Medicaid coverage for the newly eligible.

March 23, 2010
PPACA signed into law.

August 17, 2011
CMS releases proposed rule on implementing Medicaid eligibility changes under PPACA.

March 23, 2012
CMS releases final rule on implementing Medicaid eligibility changes under PPACA.

January 1, 2014
States must provide Medicaid eligibility to all individuals under age 65 up to 133 percent of the federal poverty level.

January 1, 2014
States must use the modified adjusted gross income methodology to determine Medicaid eligibility for most beneficiaries.

January 1, 2014
States must have procedures in place for a streamlined Medicaid eligibility and enrollment system and ensure it is integrated with the CHIP and exchange enrollment systems.

| 2010 | 2011 | 2012 | 2013 | 2014 |

Source: GAO analysis of CMS regulations and guidance.

CMS acknowledged that the final rule does not fully address certain aspects of the states' implementation of Medicaid expansion requirements. For example, the final rule does not address the process by which states should claim the federal match for those newly eligible individuals or how states should implement income conversion to determine whether individuals are truly newly eligible or would have been eligible for Medicaid under the state's pre-PPACA criteria. CMS is continuing to solicit comments on certain aspects of this rule and may publish further regulatory changes at a later date. For example, in June 2012, CMS released a solicitation for public input on potential methodologies for converting current eligibility standards to MAGI-equivalent standards.[14]

---

[14]CMS, Center for Medicaid and CHIP Services, *Solicitation of Public Input on Conversion of Net Income Standards to Equivalent Modified Adjusted Gross Income Standards*, (Washington, D.C., June 21, 2012).

Appendix II: States Have Taken Some Steps to Prepare for Medicaid Expansion

States Have Taken Some Steps to Prepare for Medicaid Eligibility Expansion, but Face Implementation Challenges

The six selected states in our study (Colorado, Georgia, Iowa, Minnesota, New York, and Virginia) are identifying and assessing changes that need to be made to their existing Medicaid eligibility levels and categories, and eligibility determination policies, to comply with new requirements and options for Medicaid expansion addressed in the Patient Protection and Affordable Care Act (PPACA). For example:

- Minnesota is identifying changes to eligibility levels to meet PPACA Medicaid expansion requirements. The state currently offers Medicaid to childless adults with incomes up to 75 percent of federal poverty level (FPL), but the state will need to extend coverage to those with incomes up to 133 percent of FPL. This expansion will require changes in state policies.

- Iowa is determining if it will maintain or eliminate some of its current coverage, such as the coverage it offers for individuals who are medically needy.[1] State officials are developing "Policy Option Papers" to outline necessary policy decisions and provide a list of options and recommendations for state decision makers.

- New York has identified changes to its eligibility determination processes, which currently allow a number of income exclusions that will no longer be allowed under PPACA.[2] To inform its decision making on the consolidation of eligibility categories, the state has also hired an outside research organization to compare the state's existing categories with the new consolidated categories for adults, parents, children, and pregnant women, and to outline options for ensuring alignment.

After states have determined how they need to modify their policies and processes, officials stated that various changes to eligibility policies will

---

[1] In general, states have the option of extending Medicaid coverage to the medically needy. The medically needy are individuals who fall under a Medicaid category but whose income or resources exceed applicable levels. This coverage group includes individuals who are aged, blind or disabled, members of families with children, pregnant women, and children under 21 years of age.

[2] Specifically, for the purposes of determining Medicaid eligibility, New York currently allows exclusions for certain types of income, such as child support received, room and board income, and cash assistance based on need. PPACA prohibits the use of any income exclusions for individuals whose financial eligibility will be based on modified adjusted gross income (MAGI), other than the income disregard of 5 percent of the FPL to be applied to every such individual.

require state legislative or regulatory action. State officials also said that they will need to submit amendments to their state Medicaid plans to CMS for review and approval.[3]

In an effort to streamline their eligibility and enrollment processes, all six states are taking steps to replace or upgrade their Medicaid information technology systems. These states have submitted applications to CMS for enhanced federal funding, known as advanced planning documents, to develop or upgrade their eligibility systems. State officials told us that they appreciate the enhanced funding in that it affords them an opportunity to modernize outdated eligibility and enrollment systems. Under this funding arrangement, CMS will pay the state a 90 percent match rate for the design, development and installation of Medicaid eligibility systems and a 75 percent match rate for maintenance and operations costs.[4] The six states are also issuing new requests for proposals or modifying existing contracts to secure the services of vendors with the necessary technical expertise to develop these eligibility systems.

Further, to facilitate communication and coordination between the state agencies that are developing the new eligibility systems, and direct efforts to develop new systems, the six states have formed interagency work groups. According to state officials, coordination is necessary because

[3]Some states—including Colorado, Iowa, Minnesota, New York, and Virginia—have Medicaid waivers, authorized under Section 1115 of the Social Security Act, that allow states to expand eligibility to adults who are not otherwise eligible for Medicaid. If the waiver allows a state to cover those with income above 133 percent of FPL, states also will need to decide whether to maintain the waiver or allow it to expire. For example, New York already covers childless adults up to 100 percent of FPL and parents up to 150 percent of FPL under a Section 1115 waiver. The state will need to decide whether to allow the waiver to expire, or to renew the waiver and continue coverage for parents above 133 percent of FPL.

[4]In order to qualify for the 90 percent match, states must submit an advanced planning document to CMS for approval. In approving the advanced planning document, CMS must determine that the design, development, installation, or enhancement of a state's eligibility system meets a number of standards and conditions, including seamless coordination with the health insurance exchanges. The 90 percent match is available only for costs incurred after April 19, 2011, and before December 31, 2015. Beginning April 19, 2011, states may also qualify for a 75 percent match for the operation of eligibility systems that continue to meet applicable standards and conditions. This enhanced match is not available for systems that do not meet these requirements by December 31, 2015. See, CMS, *Federal Funding for Medicaid Eligibility Determination and Enrollment Activities*, Final Rule, 76 Fed. Reg. 21950 (Apr. 19, 2011).

these systems are often used for multiple state programs, and must interface with state exchanges. These work groups often include representatives from the state Medicaid agency, state agencies responsible for other public assistance programs that use the same eligibility system, the state's office of information technology, and the entity responsible for developing the state's health benefit exchange.

States Reported That the Need for Additional Guidance and Other Challenges Could Affect Their Ability to Meet Implementation Deadlines

State officials we interviewed said they need additional federal guidance in several areas to address certain requirements under PPACA, including using MAGI to determine an applicant's Medicaid eligibility,[5] converting current net-income levels to MAGI-equivalent levels,[6] and integrating with the federal data hub.[7] CMS is taking action to issue regulations, guidance, and other types of assistance to states to support the implementation of these new requirements.

Eligibility determination. Most state officials indicated that they need additional guidance on using MAGI to determine an applicant's eligibility, under different scenarios involving household income levels, sources of income, and household composition. In March 2012, CMS issued a final rule on Medicaid eligibility and subsequently hosted a webinar that provided states with guidance for determining household income and composition under various scenarios. For example, the final rule provided a scenario for how states would determine household composition and income in the event that a taxpayer claims an adult as a dependent who is not expected to file a tax return. In addition, the webinar provided examples for determining eligibility under scenarios that involved variations in income for one-parent, two-parent, and multi-generational households. State officials said that while this guidance has been helpful, they need additional guidance to capture the range of possible scenarios that can arise in determining eligibility. For example, officials we

---

[5]MAGI is adjusted gross income, increased by certain tax-exempt interest and excluded foreign income. 26 U.S.C. § 36B(d)(2)(B).

[6]For those individuals whose eligibility will be determined using MAGI, states will need to convert their current net income standards to the new income standards under the MAGI calculation.

[7]As noted earlier, the Federal Data Services Hub is an electronic service that states will use to verify information with other federal agencies, such as an applicant's citizenship (through the Social Security Administration), immigration status (through the Department of Homeland Security), and income data (through the Internal Revenue Service).

interviewed from Colorado and Iowa noted that questions still remain about how to determine the eligibility of children who divide their time between two households with two different parents. State officials reported that until they receive sufficient guidance, moving forward with designing and implementing new eligibility determination systems will be a challenge. CMS officials told us that they are aware of the states' need for this information and plan to release additional guidance for determining eligibility in the summer of 2012.

Income conversion and submitting claims for different Federal Medical Assistance Percentage (FMAP) rates. Most state officials reported that they need additional guidance on how to convert current net income eligibility levels to MAGI-equivalent levels, to be able to distinguish applicants who will be newly eligible following the expansion from those who were previously eligible under the state's Medicaid program prior to the expansion. This is important because states will receive different matching rates for newly eligible and previously eligible adults, and need to know how to assign the appropriate FMAP rate. Since 2011, CMS has been working on a pilot effort with the RAND Corporation, the State Health Access Data Assistance Center, and 10 states[8] to identify MAGI income conversion option methodologies for claiming the appropriate FMAP rate. CMS officials indicated that this effort is ongoing and that additional publications—including regulations and technical assistance—will be forthcoming in 2012. For example, in June 2012, CMS released a solicitation for public input on potential methodologies for converting current eligibility standards to MAGI-equivalent standards.[9]

System integration with the federal data hub. State officials said they need additional guidance to determine how their systems will interface with the federal hub, the types of information they will be able to access, and whether they will be able to retain this information for quality assurance purposes. For example, some state officials we interviewed told us there is still uncertainty about the kind of information that the Internal Revenue Service will provide for verifying applicant income. This

---

[8]The 10 states included in the pilot project are: Arizona, California, Indiana, Nebraska, New Hampshire, New York, Oregon, Tennessee, Virginia, and West Virginia.

[9]Center for Medicaid and CHIP Services Informational Bulletin, *Solicitation of Public Input on Conversion of Net Income Standards to Equivalent Modified Adjusted Gross Income Standards* (Baltimore, MD, June 21, 2012).

information is important because the federal data hub will serve as a primary data source for verifying applicant information related to income and citizenship. States need to know what data will be available through the hub in order to design and implement eligibility verification. In response to questions about the status of this guidance, CMS officials said they have been working with the other federal agencies involved in providing data through the federal hub, and that the agency is close to releasing additional guidance.

In addition to federal guidance, states reported that several state-level operational issues may also challenge their ability to meet Medicaid expansion and system development deadlines. These issues include:

Lengthy procurement processes. Some state officials we interviewed said that states must follow procurement processes to secure contractors to manage the development of new eligibility systems, which can take months to complete. The length of time can be exacerbated by delays in the approval of necessary documentation, such as advanced planning documents and requests for proposals, at the federal or state level. For example, officials from Virginia reported that once all necessary documentation has been approved at the federal and state level, a request for proposal is released, and a contract is awarded, the state will likely have less than 12 months remaining to work with a vendor to implement a new system.

Complexity of developing new systems. Some state officials also reported that they must manage the complexity of developing and transitioning to a new eligibility system, which may take years to fully complete. For example, officials from New York reported that they must ultimately replace two outdated eligibility systems that are used for different parts of the state. In attempting to create a seamless operation, officials said that continuing to operate the existing program while simultaneously trying to develop and migrate to a new system will be challenging.

Coordination of multiple programs and systems. Some state officials said that their eligibility systems can be used to manage eligibility and enrollment for multiple public assistance programs, in addition to Medicaid. In these situations, developing and implementing a new eligibility system becomes significantly more complicated because states must manage the transition of multiple programs to a new system. For example, officials from Colorado reported that they share an eligibility system among multiple departments—including the state's Department of

Health Care Policy and Financing and the Department of Human Services. The state must determine how the new systems will accommodate the needs of these departments, and which components of the broader system modernization effort will take priority.

Resource limitations. Understanding and implementing eligibility and system changes required by PPACA have placed new demands on state agencies that face limitations on staff resources. For example, officials from Georgia reported that due to a recent decline in the number of available staff, the state Medicaid agency has a limited pool of staff to plan and manage large projects. At the same time that staff are preparing to comply with the Medicaid eligibility policy and system changes required by PPACA, they are also managing several other major procurements and a large Medicaid program redesign project.

To ensure key system changes are in place before 2014, state officials told us that they plan to use a phased approach to implementation. For example, in some states, this approach will focus first on ensuring that new systems are capable of determining Medicaid eligibility for applicants using MAGI beginning in 2014, while the integration of other public assistance programs is planned for later stages. Further, state officials told us that to help supplement existing staff resources, states are using vendors, consultants, and external organizations to access additional assistance and expertise.

Appendix III: States Expect Some Budgetary Impacts from Expanding Medicaid, and Expressed a Need for Additional Guidance

States Expect Some Budgetary Impacts from Expanding Medicaid, and Expressed a Need for Additional Guidance

Our survey found that across fiscal years 2012 to 2020, the majority of state budget directors believe that three aspects of Medicaid expansion will contribute to costs: (1) the administration for managing Medicaid enrollment, (2) the acquisition or modification of information technology systems to support Medicaid, and (3) enrolling previously eligible but not enrolled individuals in Medicaid (as shown in fig. 2).

Figure 2: State Budget Director Views on Fiscal Implications of Medicaid Expansion Aspects

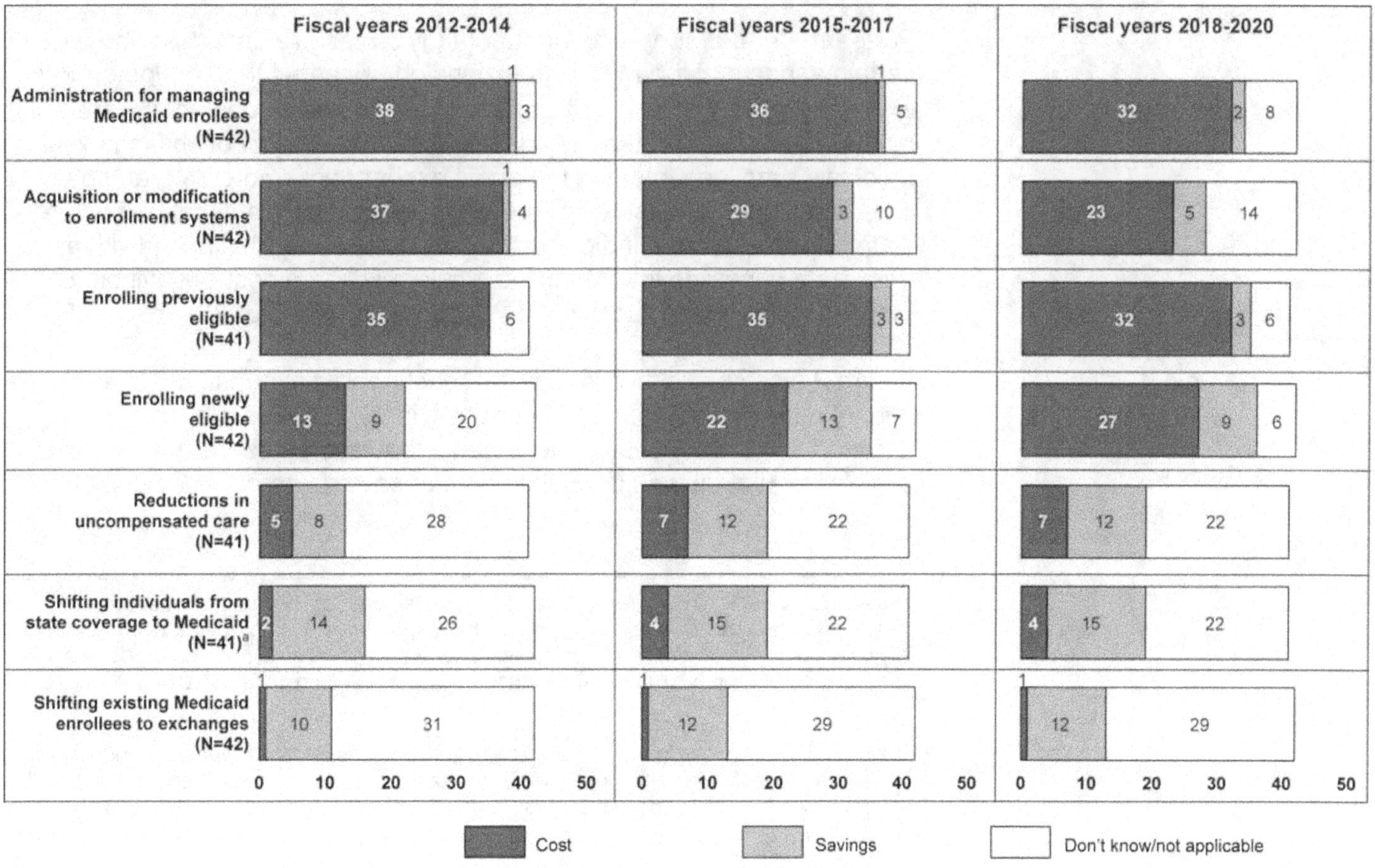

Source: GAO analysis of survey responses from state budget directors.

Note: The "N" in the graphic above refers to the total number of survey respondents.

[a]While 42 state budget officers responded to the survey question of whether shifting individuals from state coverage to Medicaid contributed a cost or savings in fiscal years 2012 through 2014, 41 budget officers responded to the question for fiscal years 2015 through 2017 and for fiscal years 2018 through 2020.

Appendix III: States Expect Some Budgetary
Impacts from Expanding Medicaid, and
Expressed a Need for Additional Guidance

Written comments provided in response to our survey, while not representative of all state budget directors, provide some insights about their views on these costs. For example, one state budget director said that in addition to the administrative costs for enrolling individuals and acquiring new information technology,[1] the state will experience other increased administrative costs for processing claims and authorizing prior claims as a result of higher Medicaid enrollment. A number of state budget directors expressed concern about costs associated with insuring individuals who are currently eligible for Medicaid but are not enrolled. A number of state budget directors said currently eligible but unenrolled individuals may now apply for Medicaid benefits due to increased outreach and penalties for those who do not purchase insurance.[2]

Furthermore, our survey found that many states are uncertain about how certain aspects of the Medicaid expansion will affect their budgets.[3] For example, across fiscal years 2012 to 2020, more than half of the state budget directors reported they did not know the impact of shifting existing Medicaid enrollees into health benefit exchanges—more so than any other expansion aspect we asked about. In addition, at least half of the state budget directors indicated they did not know if shifting individuals from state coverage into Medicaid would result in a cost or savings to their budgets across fiscal years 2012 to 2020 (see fig. 2).

Figure 2 also shows that for some aspects of the expansion, several state budget directors perceived a budget savings. For example, some reported that reductions in uncompensated care and enrolling the newly eligible population would result in budget savings across all fiscal years.

---

[1]As we noted earlier in this report, states may receive an enhanced administrative federal match—90 percent—for the design, development, and installation or enhancement of eligibility determination systems until December 31, 2015. States may also receive a 75 percent federal match for the maintenance and operations costs associated with these systems.

[2]Beginning in 2014, all United States citizens and legal residents and their dependents will be required to maintain minimum essential insurance coverage unless exempted, and will have to pay a financial penalty if they fail to maintain such coverage. PPACA § 1501(b), 124 stat. 244-49.

[3]For the purposes of this report, to characterize the 42 responses provided by state budget directors, we defined modifiers (e.g., "many") to quantify their responses as follows: "a few" or "a number of" refers to 8 or fewer responses, "several" or "some" refers to 9 to 20 responses, "many" or "more than half" refers to 21 to 31 responses, and "nearly all" refers to 32 or more responses.

Appendix III: States Expect Some Budgetary
Impacts from Expanding Medicaid, and
Expressed a Need for Additional Guidance

Several state budget directors reported also that shifting individuals from state funded coverage to Medicaid would result in budget savings for all fiscal years. However, as noted in figure 2, over half as many reported that they did not know whether this aspect would contribute costs or savings to their budgets.

States Reported That Their Fiscal Capacity and Share of Medicaid Expenditures Challenge Their Implementation of the Medicaid Expansion

Our survey asked state budget directors about their views on challenges that may affect their implementation of Medicaid expansion. Nearly all of the state budget directors reported that fiscal capacity and the state's share of Medicaid expenditures will be very or moderately challenging to implementing Medicaid expansion. Regarding other budget factors we asked about, nearly all states reported that federal funding for Medicaid expansion will be very or moderately challenging within the time period, of fiscal years 2017 to 2020, when the federal matching rate for the newly eligible enrollees will gradually decline from 95 percent to 90 percent.[4] Further, as shown in table 2, many states reported they did not know the impact of the local or county share of the states' Medicaid expenditures on their budgets.[5]

Table 2: State Budget Director Views on Challenges Affecting Medicaid Expansion

	Degree of challenge					
Challenge	Very	Moderately	Slightly	Not at all	Do not know/not applicable	Total
State fiscal capacity	28	4	4	2	4	**42**
State share of Medicaid expenditures	27	5	3	3	4	**42**
Local or county share of state Medicaid expenditures	3	3	5	6	24	**41**
Federal funding for Medicaid expansion implementation (fiscal years 2017 to 2020)	16	10	5	5	6	**42**

Source: GAO analysis of survey responses from state budget directors.

[4]As explained earlier, states will receive an increased federal match for newly eligible adults at 100 percent for 2014-2016, 95 percent in 2017, 94 percent in 2018, 93 percent in 2019, and 90 percent in 2020 and beyond.

[5]Some states require local or county governments to contribute to the state share of Medicaid expenditures. Of the states that require a local or county government contribution, the required contribution percentage varies and may include administrative, mental health, long term care, nursing home, and acute care costs.

Appendix III: States Expect Some Budgetary
Impacts from Expanding Medicaid, and
Expressed a Need for Additional Guidance

A Few State Budget Directors Reported CMS Guidance Was Useful While Many Reported Additional Guidance is Needed

Recognizing that the purpose of federal guidance is to help states implement Medicaid, we asked states how useful federal guidance was for developing budget estimates. As shown in table 3, a few state budget directors reported that the guidance was very or moderately useful, while most reported that the guidance was slightly or not at all useful.

Table 3: State Budget Director Views on Usefulness of CMS Guidance

Usefulness	Number of respondents
Very useful	2
Moderately useful	4
Slightly useful	20
Not at all useful	10
Don't know/not applicable	6

Source: GAO analysis of survey responses from state budget directors.

As part of our survey, we asked states what additional guidance, if any, they needed from CMS or other agencies to assist with developing budget estimates for Medicaid expansion. In response, 31 state budget directors provided written comments about what additional guidance they needed, which we have summarized:

- *Medicaid benefits packages.* A number[6] of state budget directors indicated they need additional guidance on definitions for essential and benchmark benefits for the newly eligible population.[7] This guidance would help clarify the types and parameters of coverage required for ambulatory, emergency, and laboratory services.

- *Medicaid eligibility determination.* Some state budget directors indicated they need additional guidance on Medicaid eligibility,

---

[6]For the purposes of this report, to characterize the 31 written responses provided by state budget directors, we defined modifiers (e.g., "a number of") to quantify their responses as follows: "a few" or "a number of" refers to 6 or fewer responses, "several" or "some" refers to 7 to 15 responses, "many" or "more than half" refers to 16 to 21 responses, and "nearly all" refers to 21 or more responses.

[7]Under PPACA, states are required to provide most people who become newly eligible under the Medicaid expansion with "benchmark" benefits. These benchmark benefits are the same level of benefits that must be provided to individuals signing up for exchange plans or who have coverage under individual or small group health plans, beginning in 2014.

Appendix III: States Expect Some Budgetary
Impacts from Expanding Medicaid, and
Expressed a Need for Additional Guidance

including methodologies for calculating Modified Adjusted Gross Income (MAGI) for the newly eligible, definitions for household composition and income for caretakers and persons with disabilities. CMS's final rule made some changes to selected eligibility determination provisions; however, a few state budget officers indicated that clarification is needed to refine state budget estimates.

- *Federal Medical Assistance Percentage (FMAP)*. Several state budget directors indicated they need guidance from CMS on submitting claims for the federal match for newly eligible adults and that such guidance is necessary for developing accurate budget estimates.

CMS officials indicated that the agency is planning to issue additional regulations or guidance such as operational bulletins at a later date in a number of areas, including clarification on eligibility groups, MAGI and the FMAP methodology for the newly eligible populations.

Appendix IV: Objectives, Scope, and Methodology

This appendix describes how we did our work to identify (1) states' responsibilities for implementing certain provisions under the Patient Protection and Affordable Care Act (PPACA),[1,2] (2) actions selected states have taken to prepare for the Medicaid expansion provisions of PPACA and the challenges they have encountered, and (3) states' views on the fiscal implications of the Medicaid expansion on state budget planning. To address these objectives, we reviewed relevant PPACA provisions; regulations and guidance issued by the Department of Health and Human Services (HHS), the Centers for Medicare & Medicaid Services (CMS), and information regarding Medicaid expansion published by state associations; we conducted semi-structured interviews with Medicaid officials in six states regarding the details of their current plans for implementing the expansion and we administered a web-based survey of state and U.S. territory budget directors. We also interviewed CMS officials responsible for developing and issuing regulations and guidance to states on the expansion.

Medicaid Expansion Provisions and Implementing Regulations and Guidance

To identify state responsibilities for implementing the Medicaid expansion provisions of PPACA, we identified relevant provisions of PPACA that impose new requirements related to Medicaid eligibility levels, modifications to eligibility determination systems, federal funding provided to support the expanded population, and changes to Medicaid enrollment processes to facilitate expansion. Specifically, we reviewed the following PPACA provisions:

1. eligibility for Medicaid coverage expanded to individuals with income at or below 133 percent of the federal poverty level;[3]

2. increased federal matching rates for costs associated with the newly eligible;[4]

---

[1]Pub. L. No. 111-148, 124 Stat. 119 (Mar. 23, 2010), as amended by HCERA, Pub. L. No. 111-152, 124 Stat. 1029 (Mar. 30, 2010).

[2]For purposes of this section, we refer to these provisions as the "Medicaid expansion provisions."

[3]PPACA § 2001(a)(1), 124 Stat. 271.

[4]PPACA § 2001(a)(3), 124 Stat. 272-3, as amended by PPACA §10201(c)(3)(B), 124 Stat. 918-19 and HCERA § 1201(1)(B), 124 Stat. 1051-52.

3. state options to offer Medicaid coverage to the newly eligible earlier than January 1, 2014;[5]

4. requirement that a state maintain its Medicaid eligibility standards until an exchange in the state is fully operational;[6]

5. the transition to using Modified Adjusted Gross Income—a tax-based definition of income—to determine income eligibility for medical assistance for non-elderly individuals;[7] and

6. the creation of streamlined eligibility and enrollment systems.[8]

Further, we reviewed certain implementing federal regulations and guidance, including rules, informational bulletins, State Medicaid Director and State Health Official letters, and questions and answers. Examples include the following:

- CMS, *Medicaid Program; Eligibility Changes Under the Affordable Care Act of 2010*, Final Rule and Interim Final Rule, 77 Fed. Reg. 17,144 (Mar. 23, 2012);

- HHS/USDA/CMS Letter to State Medicaid and CHIP Directors, State Exchange Grantees and Health & Human Service Directors providing additional guidance on cost allocation for state eligibility determination systems (Jan. 23, 2012);

- HHS/USDA/CMS Letter to State Medicaid & CHIP Directors, State Exchange Grantees and Health & Human Services Directors on cost allocation for state eligibility determination systems (Aug. 10, 2011);

- CMS Letter to State Medicaid Directors on maintenance of effort provisions (Aug. 5, 2011);

---

[5]PPACA § 2001(a)(4), 124 Stat. 274, as amended by PPACA § 10201(b), 124 Stat. 918.

[6]PPACA § 2001(b)(1)-(3), 124 Stat. 275-76.

[7]PPACA § 2002, 124 Stat. 279-82, as amended by HCERA §§ 1004(b), (e), 124 Stat. 1034, 1036.

[8]PPACA § 2201, 124 Stat. 289-91.

- CMS, *Medicaid Program; Federal Funding for Medicaid Eligibility Determination and Enrollment Activities*, Final Rule, 76 Fed. Reg. 21,950 (Apr. 19, 2011);

- Informational Bulletin on recent developments in Medicaid, including developing and upgrading Medicaid IT systems (Apr. 14, 2011);

- CMS Letter to State Medicaid Directors on maintenance of effort provisions (Feb. 25, 2011); and

- CMS Letter to State Health Officials/State Medicaid Directors on new option for coverage of individuals under Medicaid (Apr. 9, 2010).

In addition, we reviewed reports that summarized state responsibilities with regard to the Medicaid expansion required under PPACA from the Congressional Budget Office, Congressional Research Service, and relevant state associations, including: the Council of State Governments, National Association of Insurance Commissioners, National Association of Medicaid Directors, National Association of State Chief Information Officers, National Association of State Budget Officers, National Conference of State Legislatures, and National Governors Association.

Selected State Studies

To identify what actions states have taken to prepare for the implementation of the Medicaid expansion and what challenges they encountered, we administered semi-structured interviews with officials in state Medicaid offices in six states: Colorado, Georgia, Iowa, Minnesota, New York, and Virginia. We selected these states on the basis of:

1. the relative size of expected enrollment expansion within Medicaid,[9]

2. the state's Medicaid enrollment rates,

---

[9]This refers to the Medicaid Expansion Index, a measure of the relative size of a state's potential expansion made up of the number of uninsured adults who will be eligible for Medicaid in each state in 2014 and an estimate of the potential number of newly eligible Medicaid enrollees in each state. Values greater than 100 are higher than the national average and those less than 100 are lower than the national average. For additional information, see Leighton Ku, Ph.D., M.P.H.; Karen Jones, M.S.; Peter Shin, Ph.D., M.P.H.: Brian Bruen, M.S.; and Katherine Hayes, J.D. "The States' Next Challenge—Securing Primary Care for Expanded Medicaid Populations," *The New England Journal of Medicine*, vol. 364, no. 6 (Feb. 10, 2011).

3. geographic dispersion, and

4. whether a state expanded insurance coverage to childless adults in
   the past.

Table 4 provides information on the characteristics of the states we
selected.

Table 4: Characteristics of the Six Selected States Included in Our Review

State	Relative size of expected enrollment expansion	Whether the state expanded insurance coverage to childless adults in the past	Number of Medicaid enrollees (as of June 2010)
Colorado	109.5	No	526,200
Georgia	126.1	No	1,457,400
Iowa	82.8	Yes	407,300
Minnesota	90.4	Yes	712,700
New York	57.6	Yes	4,722,200
Virginia	108.7	No	785,700

Source: GAO analysis of information provided by the Kaiser Family Foundation Commission on Medicaid and the Uninsured and the work of Leighton Ku, Ph D., M P.H.; Karen Jones, M.S.; Peter Shin, Ph D., M P.H.: Brian Bruen, M.S.; and Katherine Hayes, J.D. "The States' Next Challenge—Securing Primary Care for Expanded Medicaid Populations," *The New England Journal of Medicine*, vol. 364, no. 6 (Feb. 10, 2011).

We conducted initial interviews in-person and by telephone between
January and March 2012, and follow-up interviews between April and
May 2012. The interview questions focused on: the states' policies and
procedures in implementing the Medicaid expansion, guidance and
technical assistance provided and needed for the implementation,
interagency efforts with state governments and other agencies to prepare
for the implementation, and communication between state officials. The
responses to the interviews are not intended to be representative of all
Medicaid offices.

In addition, we conducted interviews with officials from CMS and relevant
state associations, including the National Conference of State
Legislatures, National Association of State Budget Officers, and National
Association of Medicaid Directors.

Web Survey of State Budget Directors

To identify states' views on the fiscal implications of the Medicaid expansion on state budget planning, we developed and administered a web-based survey to state budget directors in the 50 states, the District of Columbia, and 4 U.S. territories (American Samoa, Guam, Puerto Rico, and the U.S. Virgin Islands). Using e-mail addresses provided by the National Association of State Budget Officers, we e-mailed each state budget director a link to a secure survey website, along with a unique identifier and password to control access to each state's questionnaire. Most survey questions were closed-ended, in which budget directors selected from a list of possible responses. To obtain additional narrative and supporting context, survey respondents were given multiple opportunities to provide additional open-ended comments throughout the survey.

We received completed questionnaires from 42 of the 55 entities, for an overall response rate of 76 percent. We conducted the survey from February 29, 2012, to April 10, 2012. Several days before the survey period began, we notified recipients that they would be receiving it. We also followed up via e-mail and telephone with nonrespondents several times before the survey period ended.

Estimates from our survey may be subject to errors from nonresponse, measurement, and data processing. We took steps in the design, data collection, and analysis of our survey to limit such errors.

While our survey sample included all states and territories in our target population, and is therefore not subject to errors from population coverage or sampling, 13 states and territories did not respond to the survey. In addition, not all those responding to the survey answered all survey questions. To minimize errors from nonresponse, we made multiple followup contacts with complete or partial nonrespondents throughout the survey. However, to the extent nonrespondents would have answered a particular question differently from those who did answer, our survey estimate for that question would differ from the true value that would have resulted had all states responded.

To limit the risk of measurement errors arising from deficiencies in questionnaire structure, question and answer wording, or respondent errors in reporting, our survey research specialists and staff with subject matter expertise designed the format and content of the questionnaire.

We pretested the survey with officials from one state to ensure that questions were clear, comprehensive, and unbiased, and to minimize the

burden the questionnaire placed on respondents. We also reviewed the
survey with officials from the National Association of State Budget
Officers. On the basis of these pretest results and comments, we revised
the questionnaire for clarity and content.

To limit possible data processing errors, survey response data were
checked for inconsistencies and ineligible responses. An independent
analyst checked all programs used to make edits to and analyze the
survey results.

In addition to the data from the survey provided in this report and its
appendixes, each survey question along with responses to it is presented
in GAO-12-944SP, an e-supplement to this report.

We conducted our work from June 2011 to July 2012 in accordance with
generally accepted government audit standards. Those standards require
that we plan and perform the audit to obtain sufficient, appropriate
evidence to provide a reasonable basis for our findings and conclusions
based on our audit objectives. We believe that the evidence obtained,
and the analysis conducted, provides a reasonable basis for our findings
and conclusions based on our audit objectives.

Appendix V: Comments from the Department of Health and Human Services

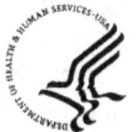

DEPARTMENT OF HEALTH & HUMAN SERVICES   OFFICE OF THE SECRETARY

_____

Assistant Secretary for Legislation
Washington, DC 20201

JUL 23 2012

Stanley J. Czerwinski
Director, Strategic Issues

Carolyn L. Yocom
Director, Health Care

U.S. Government Accountability Office
441 G Street NW
Washington, DC 20548

Dear Mr. Czerwinski and Ms. Yocom:

Attached are comments on the U.S. Government Accountability Office's (GAO) report entitled, "Medicaid Expansion: States' Implementation of the Patient Protection and Affordable Care Act" (GAO 12-821).

The Department appreciates the opportunity to review this report prior to publication.

Sincerely,

Jim R. Esquea
Assistant Secretary for Legislation

Attachment

GENERAL COMMENTS OF THE DEPARTMENT OF HEALTH AND HUMAN
SERVICES (HHS) ON THE GOVERNMENT ACCOUNTABILITY OFFICE'S (GAO)
DRAFT REPORT ENTITLED, "MEDICAID EXPANSION: STATES'
IMPLEMENTATION OF THE PATIENT PROTECTION AND AFFORDABLE CARE
ACT" (GAO-12-821)

The Department appreciates the opportunity to comment on this draft report.

The purpose of this report was to examine the actions that states are taking to implement the
Medicaid expansion under the Patient Protection and Affordable Care Act of 2010, as revised by
the Health Care and Education Reconciliation Act of 2010, hereafter referred to collectively as
the Affordable Care Act. GAO's objectives were to address the following questions: 1) What
are states' responsibilities for implementing the Medicaid expansion provisions of the Affordable
Care Act? 2) What actions have selected states taken to prepare for the implementation of the
Medicaid expansion provisions of the Affordable Care Act, and what challenges have they
encountered? 3) What are states' views on the fiscal implications of the Medicaid expansion on
state budget planning?

To address these questions, GAO surveyed states, interviewed Medicaid officials in six selected
states, sought information from state associations, and reviewed the provisions of the Affordable
Care Act. GAO also interviewed CMS officials responsible for developing and issuing
regulations and guidance on the Medicaid expansion, and reviewed the body of guidance and
other technical assistance resources that CMS has provided to states over the past 2 years. While
GAO acknowledged that CMS has been actively working to provide guidance and assistance to
states in implementing the Affordable Care Act, it concluded that states need additional
regulations and guidance in three areas: 1) application of Modified Adjusted Gross Income
(MAGI) methodology; 2) conversion of Medicaid eligibility standards; and 3) data available to
states through the Federal Data Services Hub.

Since the passage of the Affordable Care Act, the Administration has worked steadily with states
to implement the law. CMS has issued a number of guidance documents and answers to
frequently asked questions. It has hosted dozens of meetings at the national and regional levels,
conference calls, and webinars to directly engage state officials. CMS will continue to work
closely with states.

HHS and CMS acknowledge that additional guidance is needed and appreciates GAO's
acknowledgement of our efforts and planning in this regard. To assist you in finalizing the
report, below is a summary of the guidance that has been released this year and initiatives that
are underway to convey and exchange information with states regarding Affordable Care Act
implementation:

- **March 23, 2012** – Medicaid/Children's Health Insurance Program (CHIP) eligibility
  final rule published in the *Federal Register*;

- **March/April 2012** – Six webinars providing briefings of the eligibility final rule with
  approximately 500 participants per webinar;

1

**GENERAL COMMENTS OF THE DEPARTMENT OF HEALTH AND HUMAN
SERVICES (HHS) ON THE GOVERNMENT ACCOUNTABILITY OFFICE'S (GAO)
DRAFT REPORT ENTITLED, "MEDICAID EXPANSION: STATES'
IMPLEMENTATION OF THE PATIENT PROTECTION AND AFFORDABLE CARE
ACT" (GAO-12-821)**

- **March/April 2012** – Launch of State Operations and Technical Assistance (SOTA) initiative to provide individualized discussions for states with a multi-disciplinary team from CMS including representatives from the Office of the Center for Medicaid & CHIP Services (CMCS) Director, the Children and Adults Health Program Group, the Data and Systems Group, and the CMS Regional Offices. These SOTA calls will take place on a monthly basis with all 50 states;

- **April/May 2012** – Two conference calls focused specifically on how states can adopt the new eligibility standard of MAGI; two open Question and Answer sessions for states;

- **June 21, 2012** – Release of MAGI Conversion Solicitation of Public Input on two possible methodologies for converting income standards to MAGI, available at http://www.medicaid.gov/State-Resource-Center/Events-and-Announcements/Downloads/MAGI-income-conversion.pdf. This document followed a series of regular communications and data analysis work with 10 pilot states working through a contract with the RAND Corporation, CMS, and the Assistant Secretary for Planning and Evaluation;

- **July 6, 2012** – Release of proposed set of data elements for the single, streamlined application for enrollment in the Exchange, Medicaid, and CHIP, available at http://www.medicaid.gov/State-Resource-Center/Events-and-Announcements/Events-and-Announcements.html;

- **Ongoing** -- Conducting Medicaid and CHIP Learning Collaboratives with groups of 8-10 states on a range of topics. Information developed through these collaboratives is also being disseminated more broadly to all states;

- **Ongoing** -- Monthly meetings with states via Technical Advisory Groups (TAGs), such as the Children's Coverage TAG and the Eligibility TAG, which provide forums for states to receive up-to-date information and to voice questions and concerns;

- **Ongoing** – Ad hoc workgroups to discuss issues such as development of the single, streamlined application and verification and income counting rules;

- **Summer 2012** – Working with states undertaking systems modernization and offering a series of "accelerators" to help ensure that states have the resources they need to be ready for open enrollment by October 1, 2013. CMS and states have been sharing information through the Collaborative Application Lifecycle Management Tool (known as the CALT) and will be hosting numerous calls and webinars for states. These tools are complemented by the August 10, 2011, Tri-Agency Letter from CMS, the Department of Health and Human Services' Administration for Children and Families, and the Department of Agriculture providing states with information about a time-limited

2

**GENERAL COMMENTS OF THE DEPARTMENT OF HEALTH AND HUMAN
SERVICES (HHS) ON THE GOVERNMENT ACCOUNTABILITY OFFICE'S (GAO)
DRAFT REPORT ENTITLED, "MEDICAID EXPANSION: STATES'
IMPLEMENTATION OF THE PATIENT PROTECTION AND AFFORDABLE CARE
ACT" (GAO-12-821)**

exception to the cost allocation requirements set forth in the Office of Management and
Budget Circular A-87. The exception gives states the opportunity to consider the benefits
of integrating the eligibility determination functions across health and human services
programs, was effective immediately, and is available until December 31, 2015. The Tri-
Agency Letter is available at http://www.cms.gov/smdl/downloads/tri-agency.pdf.

- **Fall 2012** – CMS has been working to develop a new, electronic State Plan Amendment
  submission system, known as MACPRo, to facilitate and improve the State Plan
  Amendment review and approval process. The system is slated to become available
  beginning in January 2013, and we have been consulting with states throughout the
  development process.

As GAO notes in its report, additional rules and guidance are forthcoming and are expected to be
finalized in the near future. Specifically, as noted in the appendix to the report, CMS anticipates
issuing additional guidance on MAGI conversion in late summer 2012 and will be providing
targeted technical assistance to each state to help them think through the conversion process. It
is also working to develop final rules regarding the computation of the Federal Medical
Assistance Percentage (FMAP), based on the August 2011 Notice of Proposed Rulemaking
(76 FR 51148) and anticipate issuing a final FMAP rule in 2012. Additionally, CMS is
developing a series of operational guidance "bulletins" to assist states in applying the policies
and procedures discussed in the eligibility final rule.

Importantly, the Supreme Court's June 28, 2012 decision on the Affordable Care Act allows
states to make their own decisions about whether to undertake the Medicaid eligibility expansion
concerning certain adults without jeopardizing their pre-existing programs. There is no deadline
for a state to decide to undertake the Medicaid eligibility expansion. A state can receive extra
funding for Medicaid IT costs, even if it has not yet decided whether to expand Medicaid
eligibility, as long as it is modernizing its eligibility systems. And, if a state ultimately decides
not to undertake the eligibility expansion, it will not have to pay those resources back. More
guidance will be issued in the year and a half before the Medicaid eligibility expansion begins.

Coverage under the Medicaid eligibility expansion is completely paid for by the federal
government in the first three years, and the federal government will cover at least 90 percent of
these costs in the years thereafter. We believe that these resources, and our rules and guidance,
in addition to the interactive opportunities we continue to provide states, will enable states to
implement the Medicaid eligibility expansion in an effective manner.

GAO's report is a helpful resource for purposes of targeting our ongoing technical assistance
implementation efforts with states. We look forward to working with GAO on this and other
issues. Thank you for the opportunity to comment.

3

Appendix VI: GAO Contacts and Staff Acknowledgments

GAO Contacts

Stanley J. Czerwinski, Director, Strategic Issues, (202) 512-6806 or czerwinskis@gao.gov

Carolyn L. Yocom, Director, Health Care, (202) 512-7114 or yocomc@gao.gov

Staff Acknowledgments

In addition to the contacts named above, Michelle Sager, Acting Director; Brenda Rabinowitz, Assistant Director; Walter Ochinko, Assistant Director; Carl Ramirez, Assistant Director; Sandra Beattie, Analyst-in-Charge; Amy Bowser; Kisha Clark; Robert Gebhart; Catherine Hurley; Adam Miles; Cynthia Saunders; Hemi Tewarson; and Ann Tynan made key contributions to this report.

GAO's Mission	The Government Accountability Office, the audit, evaluation, and investigative arm of Congress, exists to support Congress in meeting its constitutional responsibilities and to help improve the performance and accountability of the federal government for the American people. GAO examines the use of public funds; evaluates federal programs and policies; and provides analyses, recommendations, and other assistance to help Congress make informed oversight, policy, and funding decisions. GAO's commitment to good government is reflected in its core values of accountability, integrity, and reliability.
Obtaining Copies of GAO Reports and Testimony	The fastest and easiest way to obtain copies of GAO documents at no cost is through GAO's website (www.gao.gov). Each weekday afternoon, GAO posts on its website newly released reports, testimony, and correspondence. To have GAO e-mail you a list of newly posted products, go to www.gao.gov and select "E-mail Updates."
Order by Phone	The price of each GAO publication reflects GAO's actual cost of production and distribution and depends on the number of pages in the publication and whether the publication is printed in color or black and white. Pricing and ordering information is posted on GAO's website, http://www.gao.gov/ordering.htm. Place orders by calling (202) 512-6000, toll free (866) 801-7077, or TDD (202) 512-2537. Orders may be paid for using American Express, Discover Card, MasterCard, Visa, check, or money order. Call for additional information.
Connect with GAO	Connect with GAO on Facebook, Flickr, Twitter, and YouTube. Subscribe to our RSS Feeds or E-mail Updates. Listen to our Podcasts. Visit GAO on the web at www.gao.gov.
To Report Fraud, Waste, and Abuse in Federal Programs	Contact: Website: www.gao.gov/fraudnet/fraudnet.htm E-mail: fraudnet@gao.gov Automated answering system: (800) 424-5454 or (202) 512-7470
Congressional Relations	Katherine Siggerud, Managing Director, siggerudk@gao.gov, (202) 512-4400, U.S. Government Accountability Office, 441 G Street NW, Room 7125, Washington, DC 20548
Public Affairs	Chuck Young, Managing Director, youngc1@gao.gov, (202) 512-4800 U.S. Government Accountability Office, 441 G Street NW, Room 7149 Washington, DC 20548